Blood Type

AB-Positive Diet Book

Complete Guide to Delicious Recipes for Your Blood Type Optimal Health and Wellness

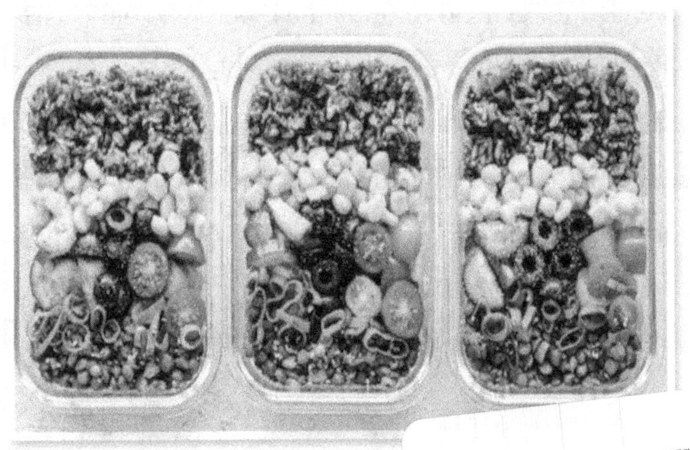

Nancy C. Hazel

Disclaimer

The information and recipes provided in this cookbook are intended for general informational purposes only. The author and publisher are not responsible for any adverse effects resulting from the use or misuse of the content contained herein. Readers are advised to consult with a qualified healthcare professional before making significant dietary changes.

Table of Contents

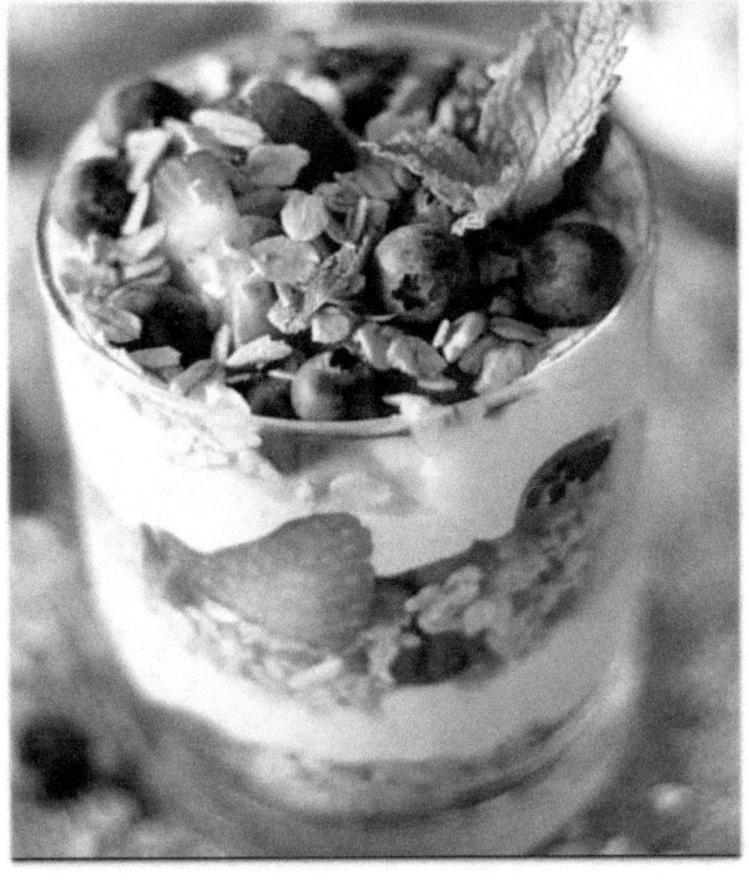

BLOOD TYPE AB *-Positive* DIET BOOK

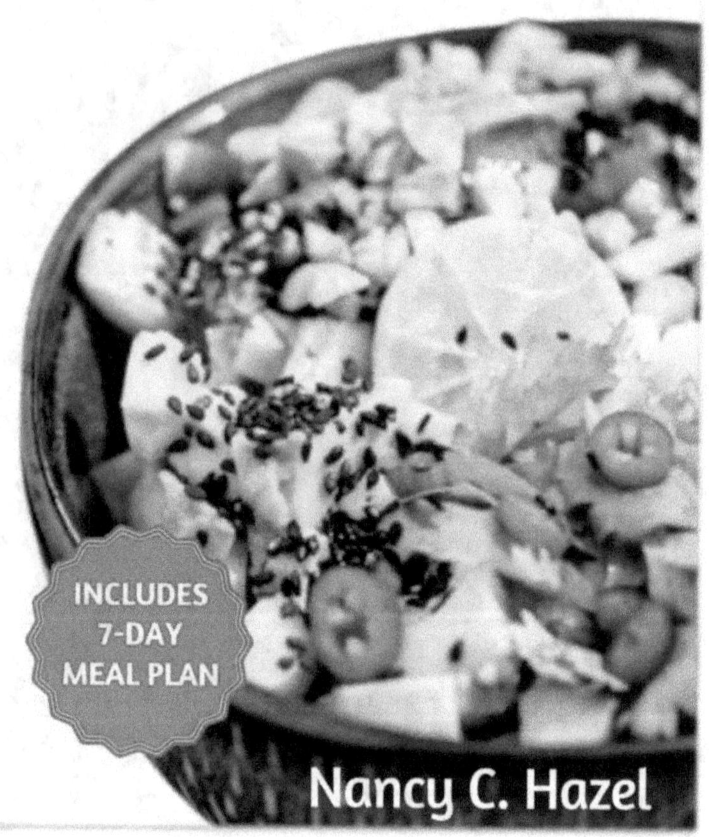

Introduction

Have you ever wondered why some foods leave you feeling energized, while others drag you down? The answer might lie in your blood type! As an AB Positive individual, you have a unique digestive system and metabolic profile that responds differently to different foods.

Welcome to a journey that goes beyond the ordinary boundaries of traditional diets. In the pages that follow, you are about to embark on a personalized odyssey designed exclusively for individuals with blood type AB positive. This is not just a cookbook; it's a guide to revolutionize the way you nourish your body, stimulate your taste buds, and enhance your overall well-being.

Given that every blood type has different dietary needs, this book has been carefully designed to meet the particular needs of those with blood type AB positive. As you explore these pages, you will find delectable recipes as well as a comprehensive approach to healthy living that is in perfect harmony with the genetic makeup of your body.

Your blood type is more than just a classification; it holds the key to a personalized and tailored approach to nutrition.

The foundation of the Blood Type AB Positive Diet is the idea that, depending on our blood type, our bodies react differently to different foods, and that, when we adjust our diet accordingly, we can achieve optimal health. This method is a lifestyle shift that can significantly enhance your digestion, energy levels, and general vigor; it's not just a fad.

You will discover a wide variety of carefully selected dishes in the upcoming chapters that will not only entice your palate but also meet the specific requirements of blood type AB positive individuals. Every meal, from tasty breakfast options to filling lunches and dinners, and even tasty snacks, is carefully crafted with attention to flavor, nutrition, and the specific requirements of your blood type.

This book extends beyond the kitchen, offering lifestyle tips and insights to help you embrace a holistic approach to healthy living. We'll explore the importance of mindful eating, exercise that complements your blood type, and the significance of adequate rest. Your path to robust health is about cultivating a balanced lifestyle that complements your own biological composition, not just what you put on your plate.

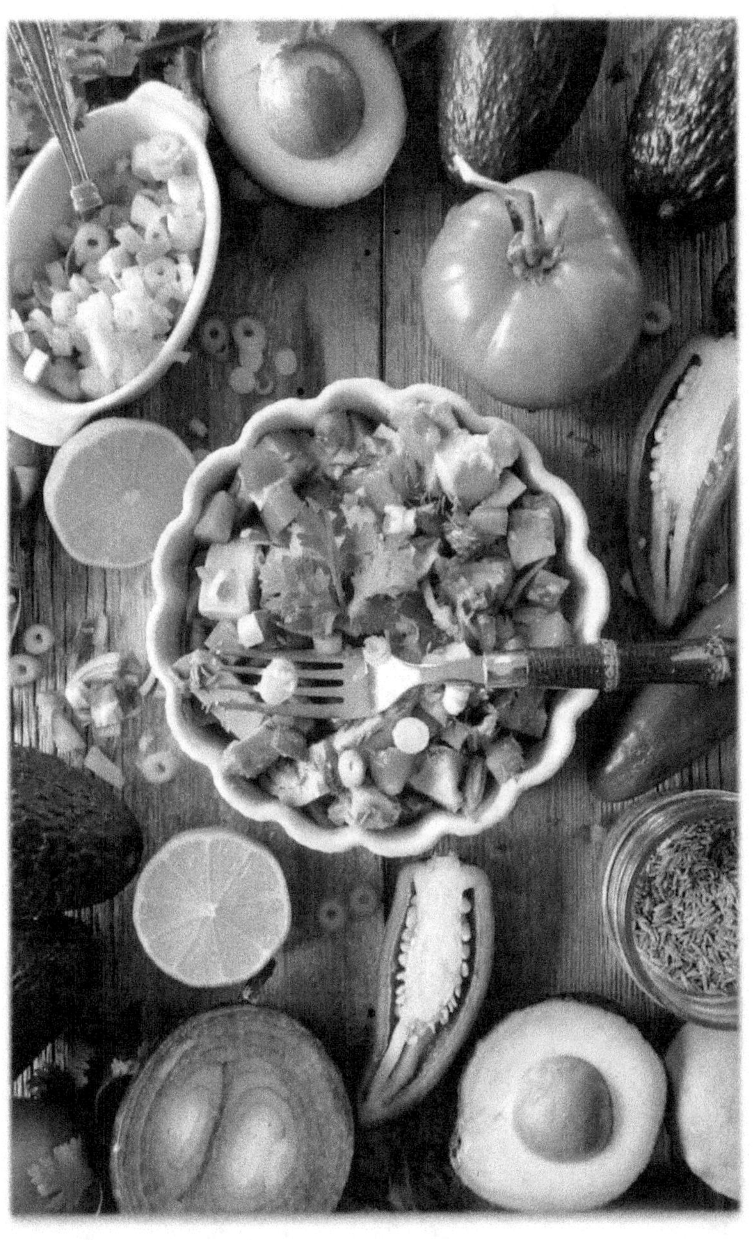

Understanding Blood Type AB Diet

Gaining knowledge about the Blood Type AB Diet serves as a compass to lead you to a more vibrant and healthy lifestyle. As individuals with blood type AB positive, you possess a unique genetic makeup that influences how your body responds to different foods. This section aims to unravel the intricacies of the Blood Type AB Diet, providing you with insights into the foods that harmonize best with your physiology. Knowing your blood type will enable you to make dietary decisions that are in line with your body's natural needs, from the importance of particular proteins to the effects of carbohydrates.

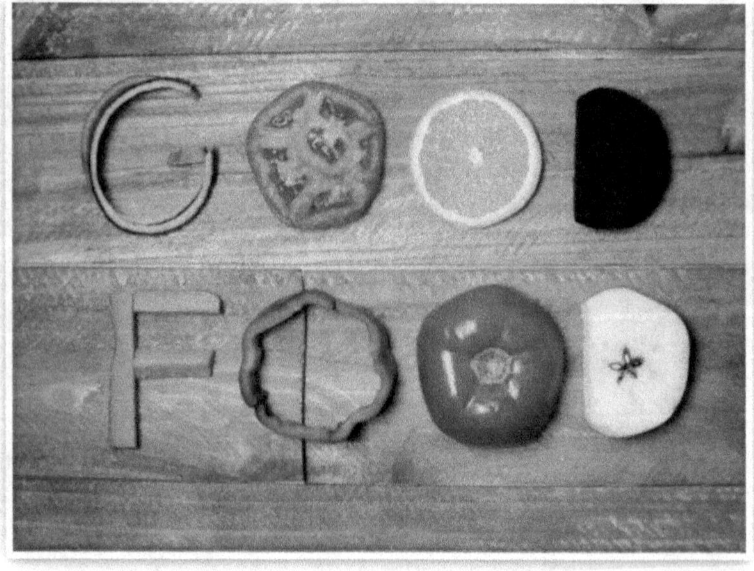

Advantage of Eating According to your Blood Type AB

Adopting the Blood Type AB Positive Diet is not only a gastronomic decision; it's a decision that will revolutionize your general health. By aligning your dietary habits with your blood type, you unlock a myriad of benefits that extend beyond the realm of taste.

1. Optimized Digestion: Eating to suit your blood type encourages effective digestion, which lowers the risk of pain and bloating. Discover a renewed sense of comfort after meals, allowing you to savor the pleasures of eating without compromise.

2. Sustained Energy Levels: Unlock the secret to sustained energy throughout the day. Eating meals that suit your blood type will give you a more consistent and long-lasting energy source, preventing weariness and promoting an active lifestyle.

3. Weight Control: There is no one-size-fits-all method for managing weight when it comes to the Blood Type AB Diet. For individuals with blood type AB positive, it acknowledges the particular elements that affect weight and provides a tailored approach to reaching and maintaining a healthy weight.

4. Enhanced Immune Function: Nourishing your body in accordance with your blood type can bolster your immune system. Discover the potential for increased resistance to illnesses and a strengthened defense against common health challenges.

5. Overall Well-Being: Beyond the physical benefits, eating according to your blood type can contribute to improved mental clarity and emotional balance. Feel a complete sense of well-being that flows from the plate into your entire existence.

As you work through the recipes and advice in this book, keep in mind that the advantages go well beyond food. Embrace the Blood Type AB Diet as a means of improving your life and your diet in order to become a healthier, more energetic version of yourself.

Chapter 1: The Basics of Blood Type AB Positive Diet

Understanding the fundamentals of the Blood Type AB Positive Diet is the first step to unlocking a harmonious relationship between your unique genetic makeup and the food you eat. This section provides an extensive summary overview of the characteristics, traits, nutritional needs, and challenges specific to individuals with blood type AB positive.

Characteristics and Traits of AB Positive Type

Known as the **"universal recipients,"** those who are AB positive blood type exhibit an intriguing combination of traits from blood types A and B. Beyond blood compatibility, this hybrid nature affects many facets of health, personality, and susceptibility to specific conditions.

1. Open-mindedness: Individuals with blood type AB positive are frequently described as having an adaptive and open-minded outlook on life, which is indicative of their blood type's flexibility.

2. Empathetic tendencies: Similar to the inclusive traits of both blood types A and B, there is a propensity for increased empathy and the capacity to comprehend many points of view.

3. Balanced outlook: Blood type AB positive people typically have a well-rounded outlook on life, balancing the characteristics of blood types A and B.

Knowing these characteristics is the first step in creating a food plan that suits the particular requirements of your blood type AB positive.

Nutritional Needs and Challenges

Recognizing the advantages and disadvantages of having blood type AB positive is essential when navigating the food landscape. Here's an overview of the dietary requirements and potential challenges:

1. Balanced Diet Emphasis: Blood type AB positive individuals thrive on a balanced diet that incorporates elements from both blood types A and B. This consists of an assortment of nutritious grains, fruits, and vegetables, as well as lean proteins.

2. Protein Considerations: Lean fish, chicken, and tofu are better options for blood type AB positive individuals than heavier meats, even though including a modest quantity of animal protein is still advantageous.

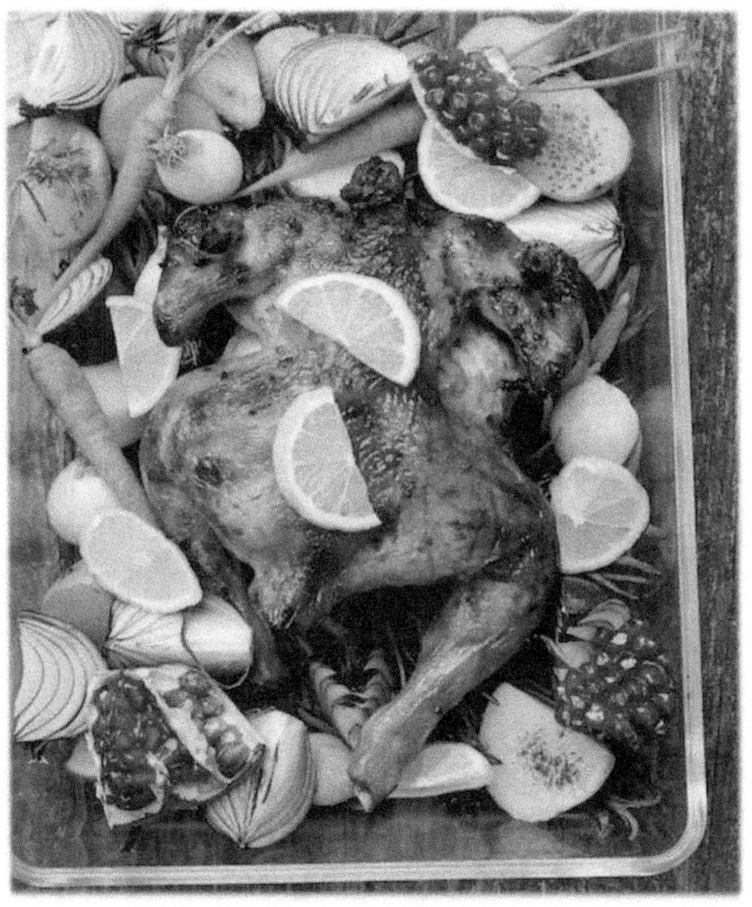

3. Digestive Sensitivity: Blood type AB positive individuals may be sensitive to some meals, especially those that include dairy or gluten. For digestion to function at its best, these sensitivities must be identified and addressed.

4. Mindful Consumption: Adopting mindful eating habits might further improve the general well-being of those with blood type AB positive by embracing the empathic and open-minded features associated with this blood type.

Understanding the fundamentals of the Blood Type AB Positive Diet will provide you the knowledge you need to choose a diet that will suit your particular genetic makeup. This basis lays the groundwork for the enticing dishes and tailored advice you may expect in the upcoming chapters. Embrace the journey towards a healthier, more vibrant lifestyle tailored to the nuances of your blood type AB positive.

Chapter 2: Foods to Embrace and Food to Avoid

Foods to Embrace on the Blood Type AB Positive Diet

Adopt a diet specific to your blood type to maximize your health potential. This is a thorough guide on foods that are beneficial to individuals with blood type AB positive:

1. Proteins for Blood Type AB Positive:

- **Lean Meats:** Incorporate foods that are high in protein without overburdening your digestive system, such as poultry, turkey, and seafood.

- **Tempeh and Tofu:** Plant-based proteins derived from soy products are great options, offering a variety of nutrients.

2. Healthy Fruits and Vegetables:

- **Dark Leafy Greens:** Spinach, kale, and Swiss chard are rich in vitamins and minerals, supporting overall well-being.

- **Berries:** Figs, cherries, and blueberries offer natural sweetness and antioxidants without upsetting the stomach.

3. Whole Grains and Legumes:

- **Quinoa:** A versatile and protein-rich grain that aligns well with the blood type AB positive diet.

- **Lentils:** These legumes are a great source of fiber and protein, which helps maintain energy levels.

4. Healthy Fats and Oils:

- **Olive Oil:** Rich in heart-healthy monounsaturated fats, olive oil is a mainstay of the Mediterranean diet.

- **Avocado:** Avocados are high in good fats that promote fullness and supply vital nutrients.

5. Dairy and Alternatives:

- **Yogurt:** For gut health, choose yogurt that is high in probiotics or non-dairy milks like coconut or almond.

- **Cheese:** Certain types of cheese, particularly feta and goat, are best enjoyed in moderation.

Foods to Avoid on the Blood Type AB Positive Diet

Be mindful of the foods that might not be compatible with your blood type as you navigate your path to maximum health. Here's a guide to what to minimize or avoid:

1. Reducing Inflammatory Foods:

- **Processed Meats:** Minimize consumption of processed and cured meats, which may contribute to inflammation.

- **Refined Sugar:** Cut back on sugary treats and opt for natural sweeteners like honey or maple syrup in moderation.

2. Reducing Possible Allergens:

- **Shellfish:** Some individuals who have blood type AB positive may be allergic to some types of shellfish; be cautious and pay attention to how your body reacts.

- **Wheat:** Although there are some whole grains that are helpful, avoid consuming too much wheat since this might lead to digestive problems.

Foods Not Compatible with Blood Type AB Positive

1. High-Fat Dairy: Steer clear of full-fat dairy as excessive intake of saturated fats may not be in line with an AB positive diet.

2. Specific Legumes: Even though many legumes are healthy, consider reducing intake of lentils and kidney beans, which may pose challenges for some individuals.

Accepting these dietary guidelines gives you the ability to make decisions that are in line with your blood type. This individualized approach to eating is a celebration of the special qualities that make you, as a person with blood type AB positive, thrive in addition to being a path toward improved well-being.

Chapter 3: Meal Planning and Preparation

Take part in a gastronomic journey created just for blood type AB positive individuals, where meal preparation and planning are crucial to maximizing health and wellbeing.

Creating Balanced Meals

The foundation of the Blood Type AB Positive Diet is preparing well-balanced meals. Here's a quick tip to help you make recipes that are both tasty and nourishing:

1. Protein Focus: Make seafood, tofu, and lean meats the main ingredients of your meals.

2. Abundant Vegetables: Pile your plate with a variety of colorful vegetables, especially dark leafy greens and antioxidant-rich options.

3. Whole Grains: For long-lasting energy, incorporate whole grains that are high in nutrients, such as brown rice and quinoa.

4. Healthy Fats: Incorporate in moderation foods like almonds, avocados, and olive oil that are good sources of fat.

5. Mindful Portions: Be mindful of portion sizes to guarantee a balanced nutrient intake without overloading your system.

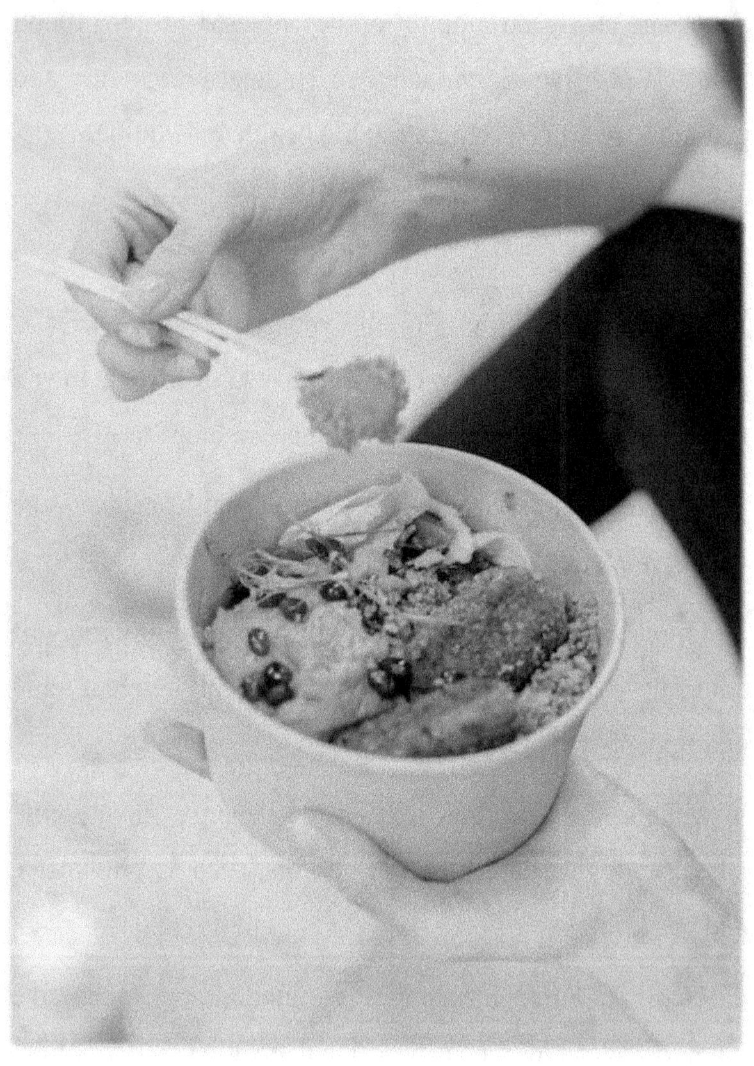

Guidelines for Grocery Shopping

Blood type AB positive meal planning success depends on purposefully navigating the aisles. Consider these tips for a fruitful grocery shopping experience:

1. List Essentials: To prevent impulsive purchases, plan your meals ahead of time and make a thorough shopping list.

2. Emphasize on Fresh: Give priority to fresh produce, lean proteins, and whole foods to fill your cart with nutrient-dense selections.

3. Check the Labels: Examine food labels closely for any components, preservatives, or hidden additives that might not be compatible with your blood type

Cooking Methods for Nutrient Retention

Use cooking methods that put health first to maintain the nutritional integrity of your ingredients:

Steaming: Gently steam vegetables to preserve their maximum nutritional content.

Sautéing: For quick and tasty cooking without compromising nutritional value, use healthy oils and moderate heat.

Grilling and Baking: Explore grilling and baking as methods to enhance the taste of lean proteins while maintaining their nutritional content.

Experiment with Herbs: For a sensory-rich meal, try different herbs and spices to enhance flavors without adding too much salt.

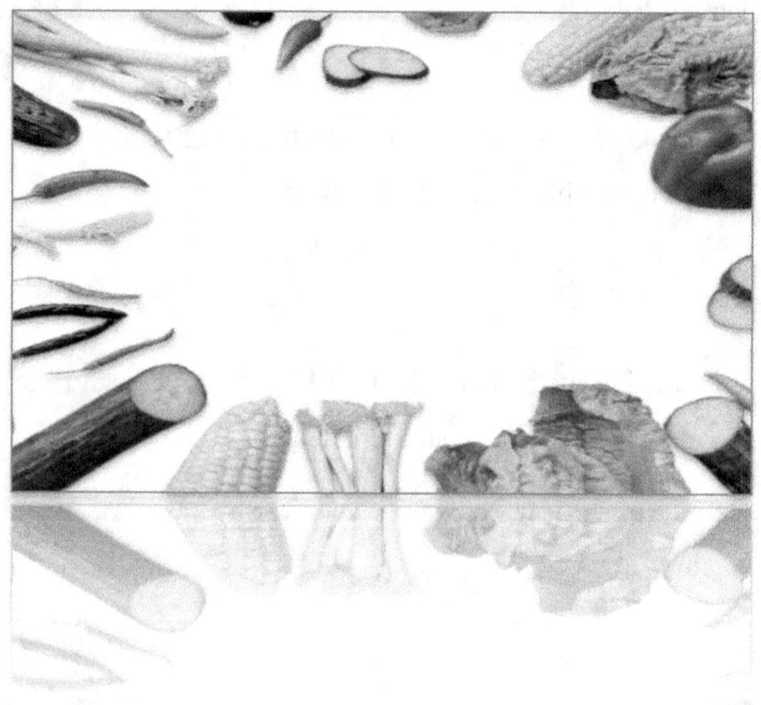

Chapter 4: Meals and Recipes Selection

Breakfast Boosters

1. Mediterranean Breakfast Wrap

Ingredients	Instructions
- 1 tortilla or whole grain wrap	1. Cover the whole grain wrap with hummus.
- 2 scrambled eggs	2. Layer cherry tomatoes, diced cucumber, sliced Kalamata olives, and scrambled eggs.
- 2 tablespoons hummus	
- 1/4 cup diced cucumber	
- 1/4 cup halved cherry tomatoes	3. Garnish with fresh parsley and fold the wrap into a delicious Mediterranean-inspired breakfast.
- Sliced Kalamata olives	
- To garnish, fresh parsley	

2. Quinoa and Berry Breakfast Bowl

Prep Time: 15 minutes (assuming quinoa is pre-cooked)

Ingredients	Instructions
- 1/2 cup of mixed berries (strawberries, raspberries, blueberries) - 1 cup cooked quinoa - 1 tablespoon chia seeds - 1 tablespoon chopped nuts (walnuts or almonds) - 1/2 cup unsweetened almond milk - 1 teaspoon honey	1. Combine cooked quinoa and mixed berries in a bowl. 2. Top the quinoa and berries with chopped almonds and chia seeds. 3. For added natural sweetness, drizzle some honey over the mixture. 4. Drizzle almond milk on top. 5. Gently combine the ingredients, then have your breakfast dish full of nutrients and protein!

3. Tofu and Spinach Scramble

Cooking Time: 10 minutes

Ingredients	Instructions
- 1/2 cup crumbled firm tofu	1. In a skillet, heat olive oil over medium heat.
- 1/4 cup halved cherry tomatoes	2. Add minced garlic and sauté until aromatic.
- 1 cup chopped fresh spinach	3. Add bell pepper, spinach, cherry tomatoes, and crumbled tofu.
- 1/4 cup red bell pepper, diced	4. Simmer until the tofu is slightly golden and the spinach begins to wilt.
- 1 minced garlic clove	5. To taste, add salt and pepper for seasoning.
- 1 tablespoon olive oil	6. Serve this plate of protein-rich scramble on a plate and get your day going!
- To taste, add salt and pepper.	

4. Blueberry and Almond Smoothie

Prep Time: 5 minutes

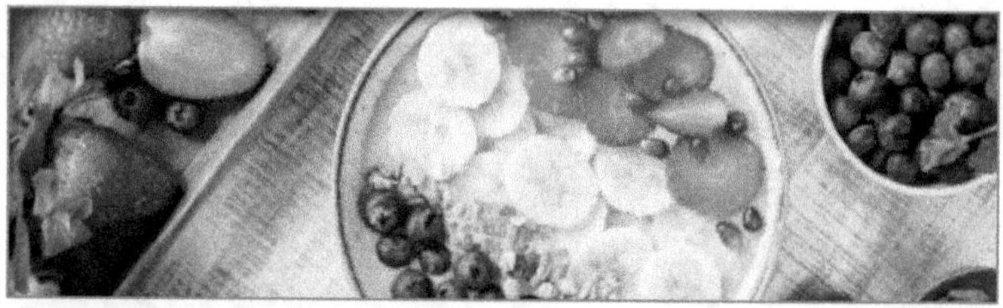

Ingredients	Instructions
- 1/2 cup (frozen or fresh) blueberries - 1 banana - 1/4 cup almond butter - 1 cup unsweetened almond milk - 1 tablespoon flaxseed - Ice cubes, if desired	1. In a blender, combine the almond milk, flaxseeds, banana, blueberries, and almond butter. 2. Blend until creamy and smooth. 3. If you want a cooler consistency, add ice cubes. 4. Transfer to a glass and enjoy this nutrient-rich, revitalizing smoothie.

5. Greek Yogurt Parfait with Mixed Fruit

Preparation Time: 7 minutes

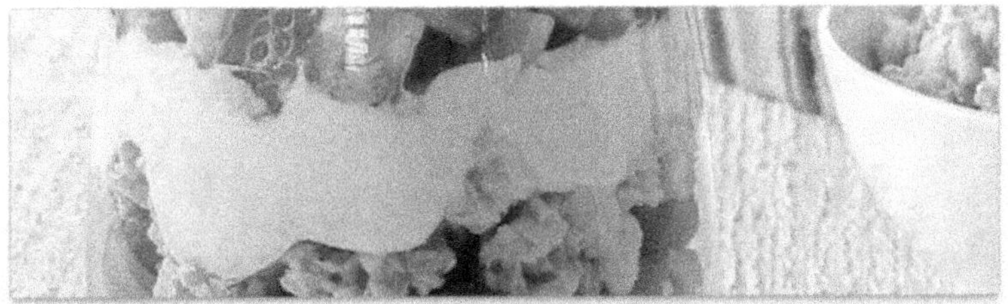

Ingredients	Instructions
- 1 cup Greek yogurt - 1/2 cup granola (ensure it's suitable for blood type AB). - 1/2 cup diced mixed fruits (apple, pineapple, and kiwi). - 1 tablespoon of honey	1. Layer Greek yogurt at the bottom of a glass or bowl. 2. Sprinkle some granola on top. 3. Top with mixed fruits. 4. For sweetness, drizzle honey over the fruits. 5. Repeat the layers again. 6. Add a granola and yogurt dollop as finishing touches.

6. Salmon and Avocado Toast

Prep Time: 10 minutes

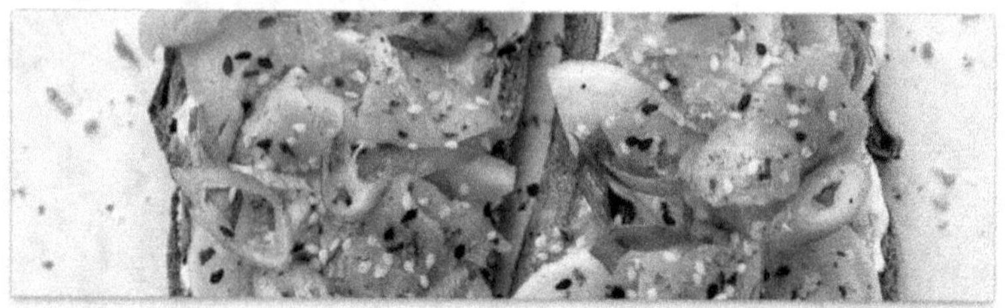

Ingredients	Instructions
- 1/2 mashed avocado	1. Lightly toast the bread slices to your desired.
- 2 slices of bread	2. Evenly spread mashed avocado on each slice.
- 100g smoked salmon	3. Top with smoked salmon and sprinkle capers on top of the salmon.
- 1 tablespoon capers	4. Season with salt and pepper to taste.
- Garnish with lemon wedges	5. Serve with lemon wedges on the side and garnish with fresh dill.
- Fresh dill for garnish	
- Salt and pepper to taste.	

7. Sweet Potato and Turkey Breakfast Hash

Prep Time: 15 minutes | Cooking Time: 20 minutes

Ingredients	Instructions
- 1/2 cup diced bell peppers (any color) - 4 ounces ground turkey - 1 medium sweet potato, peeled and chopped - 1/4 cup finely chopped red onion - 1 minced garlic clove - 1 tablespoon olive oil - Season with salt and pepper - Garnish with fresh parsley	1. Heat olive oil in a skillet over medium heat. 2. Add ground turkey and cook until it browns. Take out and place aside from the skillet. 3. In the same skillet, add more olive oil if needed, and sauté sweet potatoes until slightly crispy. 4. Add minced garlic, red onion, and diced bell peppers. Sauté the vegetables until softened. 5. Place the cooked turkey back into the skillet and toss all the ingredients. 6. Add salt and pepper for seasoning, then top with fresh parsley.

8. Salmon and Asparagus Frittata

Prep Time: 15 minutes | Cooking Time: 20 minutes

Ingredients	Instructions
- 4 eggs - 1/2 cup flaked smoked salmon - 1/2 cup chopped asparagus - 1/4 cup diced red bell pepper - 1 tablespoon freshly chopped dill - To taste, add salt and pepper - 1 tablespoon olive oil	1. Preheat the oven to 350°F (175°C). 2. Whisk eggs in a bowl and add pepper and salt to taste. 3. Heat olive oil in an oven-safe skillet over medium heat. 4. Add the red bell pepper and asparagus and sauté until slightly softened. 5. Top the vegetables with whisked eggs, smoked salmon, and freshly chopped dill. 6. Transfer the skillet to the oven and bake for 15 to 20 minutes, or until the frittata sets.

9. Buckwheat Banana Pancakes

Prep Time: 10 minutes | Cooking Time: 15 minutes

Ingredients	Instructions
- 1 ripe banana - 1/2 cup buckwheat flour - 1/2 teaspoon baking powder - 1 egg - 1/4 teaspoon cinnamon - 1/4 cup almond milk - Coconut oil for cooking	1. Combine almond milk, banana, egg, baking powder, cinnamon, and buckwheat flour in a blender. 2. Blend until smooth. If necessary, adjust the consistency with additional almond milk. 3. Heat coconut oil in a pan and pour small amounts of batter to make pancakes. 4. Cook until bubbles appear, then turn and cook the other side.

10. Chia and Mixed Berry Jam Toast

Prep Time: 15 minutes

Ingredients	Instructions
- 2 slices of whole grain bread - 2 teaspoons chia seeds - 1/2 cup of mixed berries (raspberries, blueberries, strawberries) - 1 tablespoon maple syrup or honey - Almond butter (if desired)	1. To create a jam-like consistency, combine mixed berries with chia seeds in a bowl and let it settle for 10 minutes. 2. Toast the whole grain bread slices to your desired. 3. If preferred, spread almond butter over the toasted bread. 4. Drizzle some honey or maple syrup over the toast and top with the chia and mixed berry jam.

1. Turkey and Quinoa Stuffed Peppers

Prep Time: 20 minutes | Cooking Time: 30 minutes

Ingredients	Instructions
- 4 bell peppers, halved and seeded	1. Preheat the oven to 375°F (190°C).
- 1 cup cooked quinoa	2. In a skillet, heat olive oil over medium heat.
- 8 ounces ground turkey	3. Add ground turkey and heat until it browns.
- 1/2 cup diced tomatoes	4. Add the minced garlic, red onion, and diced tomatoes. Sauté the veggies until they are tender.
- 1 minced clove garlic	5. Stir in cumin, salt, pepper, and cooked quinoa.
- 1/4 cup red onion, finely chopped	6. Stuff the turkey and quinoa mixture into the halved bell pepper.
- 1 teaspoon olive oil	7. Place the stuffed peppers in a baking dish, cover with foil, and bake for 25-30 minutes.
- 1 teaspoon cumin	
- Salt and pepper to taste	
- Fresh cilantro for garnish	

8. Before serving, garnish with fresh cilantro.

2. Lentil and Vegetable Stir-Fry

Prep Time: 15 minutes | Cooking Time: 15 minutes

Ingredients	Instructions
- 1 cup cooked lentils	1. Heat olive oil in a wok or skillet over medium-high heat.
- 1 cup broccoli florets	2. Add minced garlic and ginger and cook until aromatic.
- 1/2 cup sliced snap peas	3. Add julienned carrot, snap peas, and broccoli. Stir-fry the vegetables until softened.
- 1 julienned carrot	4. Add cooked lentils and the soy sauce, and toss to well combine.
- 2 tablespoons soy sauce	5. Cook for further 2 to 3 minutes, or until the flavors blend.
- 1 teaspoon minced ginger	6. Before serving, garnish with sesame seeds.
- 1 tablespoon olive oil	
- 2 minced garlic cloves	
- 1 tablespoon sesame seeds for garnish	

3. Grilled Chicken and Quinoa Salad

Prep Time: 20 minutes

Ingredients	Instructions
- 1 cup cooked quinoa - 6 ounces of sliced grilled chicken breast - 2 cups mixed green salad - 1/2 sliced cucumber - 1/2 cup halved cherry tomatoes - 1/4 cup crumbled feta cheese - 1 tablespoon balsamic vinegar - 2 teaspoons olive oil - To taste, add salt and pepper	1. Combine the cooked quinoa, feta cheese, cucumber, cherry tomatoes, salad greens, and grilled chicken in a big bowl. 2. Whisk together olive oil, balsamic vinegar, salt, and pepper in a small bowl. 3. Pour the salad with the dressing and gently toss to mix. 4. Serve right away as a refreshing, high-protein salad.

4. Shrimp and Vegetable Stir-Fry with Brown Rice

Prep Time: 20 minutes | Cooking Time: 15 minutes

Ingredients	Instruction
- 1 cup cooked brown rice - 8 ounces peeled and deveined shrimp - 1 cup broccoli florets - 1/2 sliced red bell pepper - 1/2 cup snow peas - 1 julienned carrot - 2 tablespoons soy sauce - 1 teaspoon sesame oil - 1 tablespoon olive oil - 1 teaspoon minced ginger - 2 minced garlic cloves - Green onions as garnish	1. Heat the sesame oil and olive oil in a wok or skillet over medium-high heat. 2. Add the minced garlic and ginger and cook until aromatic. 3. Add shrimp and stir-fry until fully cooked and pink. 4. Add julienned carrot, bell pepper, snow peas, and broccoli. Vegetables should be stir-fried until crisp-tender. 5. Add the soy sauce and whisk everything together. 6. Spoon cooked brown rice over the shrimp and vegetables stir-fried. 7. Before serving, garnish with sliced green onions.

5. Quinoa and Vegetable Buddha Bowl

Prep Time: 15 minutes

Ingredients	Instructions
- 1/2 cup rinsed and drained chickpeas	1. Combine cooked quinoa, shredded carrots, cherry tomatoes, avocado slices, and chickpeas in a bowl.
- 1/2 sliced avocado	
- 1/2 cup halved cherry tomatoes	
- 1/4 cup carrots, shredded	2. Combine the olive oil, lemon juice, salt, and pepper in a small bowl.
- 1/4 cup hummus	
- 1 tablespoon lemon juice	3. Drizzle the dressing over the bowl and add a dollop of hummus.
- 1 tablespoon olive oil	
- Season with salt and pepper	4. Add fresh parsley as garnish and enjoy this nutrient-dense Buddha Bowl.
- Garnish with fresh parsley	

6. Eggplant and Chickpea Stew

Prep Time: 15 minutes | Cooking Time: 20 minutes

Ingredients	Instruction
- 1 medium eggplant, diced - 1 can (15 ounces), rinsed and drained chickpeas - 1 cup diced tomatoes - 1/2 cup chopped red bell pepper - 1/4 cup finely chopped red onion - 2 minced garlic cloves - 1/2 teaspoon smoked paprika - 1 teaspoon cumin - 2 tablespoons olive oil - Season with salt and pepper - Garnish with fresh cilantro	1. In a pot, heat olive oil over medium heat. 2. Add diced eggplant, red onion, and minced garlic. Sauté until the eggplant begins to get tender. 3. Add the smoked paprika, cumin, diced tomatoes, red bell pepper, chickpeas, and salt and pepper. 4. Simmer until the stew thickens and the flavors combine, about 15 to 20 minutes. 5. Before serving, garnish with fresh cilantro.

7. Spinach and Mushroom Quiche

Prep Time: 20 minutes | Cooking Time: 30 minutes

Ingredients	Instruction
- 4 eggs	1. Preheat the oven to 375°F (190°C).
- 1 premade whole grain pie crust	2. In a skillet, heat olive oil over medium heat.
- 1 cup chopped spinach	3. Sauté the mushrooms and spinach until they wilt and the extra moisture drains out.
- 1/2 cup sliced mushrooms	4. Whisk eggs in a bowl and add milk, feta crumbles, sautéed spinach, and mushrooms. Add some nutmeg, salt, and pepper for seasoning.
- 1/2 cup crumbled feta cheese	5. Fill the prepared pie crust with the egg mixture.
- 1/2 cup milk (non-dairy or dairy)	6. Bake the quiche for 25 to 30 minutes, or until it sets and turns golden brown.
- 1 tablespoon olive oil	
- Salt and pepper to taste	
- Nutmeg for seasoning	

8. Thai-Inspired Chicken Lettuce Wraps

Prep Time: 15 minutes | Cooking Time: 15 minutes

Ingredients	Instruction
- 8 (butter or iceberg) lettuce leaves - 1 pound ground chicken - 1/2 cup chopped water chestnuts - 1/4 cup sliced green onions - 1/4 cup chopped cilantro - 2 tablespoons soy sauce - 1 tablespoon hoisin sauce - 1 tablespoon minced ginger - 1 minced garlic clove - 1 tablespoon lime juice - 1 tablespoon sesame oil	1. Heat sesame oil in a skillet over medium heat. 2. Add minced garlic and ginger and cook until aromatic. 3. Add ground chicken and cook it until it turns brown. 4. Stir in lime juice, soy sauce, hoisin sauce, cilantro, green onions, and water chestnuts. Cook until well mixed. 5. Spoon the chicken mixture onto lettuce leaves. 6. Roll he leaves into wraps and, if necessary, fasten with toothpicks.

9. Mediterranean Quinoa Salad

Prep Time: 15 minutes

Ingredients	Instructions
- 1 cup cooked quinoa	1. Combine cooked quinoa, cucumber, cherry tomatoes, feta cheese, olives, and red onion in a big bowl.
- 1/2 cup halved cherry tomatoes	
- 1/2 diced cucumber	
1/4 cup sliced Kalamata olives	
- 1/4 cup crumbled feta cheese	2. Combine the olive oil, balsamic vinegar, salt, pepper, and dried oregano in a small bowl.
- 1 tablespoon balsamic vinegar	
- 2 tablespoons olive oil	3. Pour the salad with the dressing and gently toss to mix.
- 2 tablespoons finely sliced red onion	
- 1 teaspoon dried oregano	4. Serve chilled as a refreshing and nutrient-packed Mediterranean salad.
- To taste, add salt and pepper.	

10. Teriyaki Salmon with Steamed Vegetables

Prep Time: 15 minutes | Cooking Time: 20 minutes

Ingredients	Instructions
- 2 salmon fillets	1. Preheat the oven to 400°F (200°C).
- 1 cup broccoli florets	2. Layer salmon fillets on a parchment paper-lined baking pan.
- 1/2 cup snap peas	3. Apply teriyaki sauce to the salmon and bake it for 15 to 20 minutes, or until cooked through.
- 1 sliced carrot	
- 2 tablespoons teriyaki sauce	4. Steam broccoli, snap peas, and sliced carrot in a steamer until crisp-tender.
- 1 tablespoon olive oil	5. In a skillet, heat olive oil over medium heat.
- Sesame seeds for garnish	6. Sauté steamed vegetables briefly and served alongside teriyaki salmon.
- Green onions for garnish	7. Add sliced green onions and sesame seeds as garnish.

1. Baked Lemon Herb Chicken

Prep Time: 15 minutes | Cooking Time: 30 minutes

Ingredients	Instruction
- 4 chicken breasts, skinless and boneless	1. Preheat the oven to 400°F (200°C).
- 2 tablespoons fresh lemon juice	2. Combine olive oil, lemon juice, minced garlic, dried thyme, dried oregano, salt, and pepper in a bowl.
- 2 tablespoons olive oil	
- 2 minced garlic cloves	3. Transfer the chicken breasts to a baking dish and pour the lemon herb mixture over it.
- 1 teaspoon oregano, dried	
- 1 teaspoon thyme, dried	4. Bake the chicken for 25 to 30 minutes, or until it is thoroughly cooked.
- Salt and pepper to taste	
- Lemon slices for garnish	5. Before serving, garnish with fresh parsley and lemon slices.
- Fresh parsley for garnish	

2. Stir-Fried Tofu with Vegetables

Prep Time: 20 minutes | Cooking Time: 15 minutes

Ingredients	Instruction
- 1 block cubed firm tofu	1. Press tofu to remove excess water and slice into cubes.
- 2 tablespoons soy sauce	2. Marinate tofu in soy sauce for 10 minutes in a bowl.
- 1 tablespoon olive oil	3. Heat olive oil in a wok or skillet over medium-high heat.
- 1 cup broccoli florets	4. Add minced ginger and garlic, and sauté until aromatic.
- 1/2 sliced red bell pepper	5. Stir in marinated tofu and cook until golden brown.
- 1/2 cup snow peas	6. Add julienned carrot, broccoli, snow peas, and red bell pepper. Vegetables should be stir-fried until crisp-tender.
- 1 julienned carrot	7. Before serving, garnish with sliced green onions and sesame seeds.
- 2 minced garlic cloves	
- 1 tablespoon minced ginger	
- 1 tablespoon sesame seeds as garnish	
- Green onions for garnish	

3. Quinoa and Black Bean Stuffed Peppers

Prep Time: 20 minutes | Cooking Time: 30 minutes

Ingredients	Instruction
- 4 bell peppers, halved and seeds removed	1. Turn the oven on to 375°F, or 190°C.
- 1 cup cooked quinoa	2. In a skillet, heat olive oil over medium heat.
- 1 can (15 ounces) drained and rinsed black beans	3. Add diced tomatoes, red onion, and minced garlic. Cook veggies until tender.
- 1 cup tomatoes, diced	4. Add black beans, cumin, chili powder, salt, and pepper along with cooked quinoa.
- 1/2 cup finely chopped red onion	5. Stuff the black bean and quinoa mixture into halved bell peppers.
- 1 clove garlic, minced	6. Put the filled peppers in a baking dish, cover it with foil, and bake it for 25 to 30 minutes.
- 2 tablespoons olive oil	7. Before serving, garnish with fresh cilantro.
- 1 teaspoon cumin	
- 1/2 teaspoon chili powder	
- Salt and pepper to taste	
- Fresh cilantro for garnish	

4. Lemon Garlic Shrimp with Zucchini Noodles

Prep Time: 15 minutes | Cooking Time: 10 minutes

Ingredients	Instruction
- 1 pound peeled and deveined shrimp - 4 medium zucchini, spiralized into noodles - 2 tablespoons olive oil - 3 minced cloves of garlic - 2 tablespoons fresh lemon juice - 1 teaspoon lemon zest - 1/4 teaspoon red pepper flakes, if desired - To taste, add salt and pepper - Fresh parsley for garnish - Grated Parmesan cheese (optional)	1. In a large skillet, heat olive oil over medium heat. 2. Add minced garlic and sauté until aromatic. 3. Add shrimp and cook until pink and opaque. 4. Add the red pepper flakes, lemon zest, and lemon juice. Stir in pepper and salt for seasoning. 5. Add zucchini noodles and mix until they are well warm. 6. Before serving, garnish with grated Parmesan cheese and fresh parsley, if preferred.

5. Mediterranean Baked Cod

Prep Time: 15 minutes | Cooking Time: 20 minutes

Ingredients	Instruction
- 2 tablespoons olive oil	1. Set the oven's temperature to 400°F (200°C).
- 1 tablespoon lemon juice	2. Combine olive oil, lemon juice, minced garlic, dried basil, dried oregano, paprika, salt, and pepper in a small bowl.
- 4 cod fillets	
- 2 minced garlic cloves	
- 1 teaspoon oregano, dried	3. Layer cod fillets on a baking tray and drizzle with the mixture of olive oil.
- 1/4 teaspoon paprika	
- 1/2 teaspoon dried basil	4. Place Kalamata olives and cherry tomatoes around the cod fillets.
- Salt and pepper to taste	
- Cherry tomatoes for garnish	5. Bake the cod for 15 to 20 minutes, or until it is thoroughly cooked.
- Kalamata olives for garnish	
- Fresh parsley for garnish	6. Before serving, garnish with fresh parsley.

6. Vegetable and Chickpea Coconut Curry

Prep Time: 15 minutes | Cooking Time: 20 minutes

Ingredients	Instruction
- 1 can (15 ounces) rinsed and drained chickpeas - 1/2 cup cauliflower florets - 1 cup broccoli florets - 1 sliced carrot - 1/2 sliced red bell pepper - 1/2 cup snap peas - 1 can (14-ounce) coconut milk - 2 tablespoons red curry paste. - 1 tablespoon olive oil - 1 tablespoon soy sauce - Cooked brown rice for dishing - Fresh cilantro for garnish	1. Heat the olive oil in a wok or big skillet over medium-high heat. 2. Add snap peas, red bell pepper, broccoli, cauliflower, and carrot. Sauté until the vegetables are crisp-tender. 3. Toss in the soy sauce and red curry paste, evenly coating the veggies. 4. Add the coconut milk, bring to a simmer, and cook for a further 5 minutes. 5. Serve the vegetable and chickpea coconut curry over cooked brown rice. 6. Before serving, garnish with fresh cilantro.

7. Turkey and Spinach Stuffed Mushrooms

Prep Time: 20 minutes | Cooking Time: 25 minutes

Ingredients	Instruction
- 16 large mushrooms with stems removed	1. Preheat the oven to 375°F (190°C).
- 1/2 pound ground turkey	2. In a skillet, heat olive oil over medium heat.
- 1 cup chopped spinach	3. Add red onion and minced garlic and sauté until tender.
- 1/4 cup finely chopped red onion	4. Add ground turkey and heat it until it browns. Add chopped spinach and stir until it wilts.
- 2 minced garlic cloves	5. Add salt, pepper, and dried oregano for seasoning.
- 1/4 cup crumbled feta cheese	6. Stuff the turkey and spinach mixture into each mushroom.
- 1 tablespoon olive oil	7. Transfer the filled mushrooms to a baking tray and top with feta cheese crumbles.
- 1 teaspoon dried oregano	
- To taste, add salt and pepper.	

8. Bake for 20-25 minutes or until mushrooms are softened.

8. Lemon Herb Quinoa with Grilled Shrimp

Prep Time: 15 minutes | Cooking Time: 10 minutes

Ingredients	Instruction
- 1 pound peeled and deveined shrimp - 2 teaspoons olive oil - 1 tablespoon fresh lemon juice - 1 cup cooked quinoa - 1 teaspoon dried basil - 1 teaspoon dried thyme - 1/2 teaspoon garlic powder - Lemon wedges for serving - Fresh parsley for garnish - Salt and pepper to seasoning	1. Combine cooked quinoa, garlic powder, olive oil, fresh lemon juice, dried thyme, dried basil, and salt and pepper in a bowl. 2. Toss shrimp in another bowl and sprinkle with salt, pepper, and olive oil. 3. Grill shrimp per side until they are pink and fully cooked, for about 2 to 3 minutes. 4. Serve the grilled shrimp over the lemon herb quinoa. 5. Add fresh parsley and lemon wedges as garnish.

9. Baked Sweet Potato and Chickpea Falafel

Prep Time: 20 minutes | Cooking Time: 25 minutes

Ingredients	Instruction
- 1 can (15 ounces) of rinsed and drained chickpeas - 2 medium sweet potatoes, peeled and grated - 1/4 cup finely chopped red onion - 2 minced garlic cloves - 1/4 cup chopped fresh cilantro - 1/2 teaspoon paprika - 1 teaspoon ground cumin - 1 teaspoon ground coriander - To taste, add salt and pepper. - 2 tablespoons olive oil. - Tahini sauce for dressing	1. Preheat the oven to 400°F (200°C). 2. Combine grated sweet potatoes, chickpeas, red onion, minced garlic, paprika, cumin, coriander, cilantro, and salt and pepper in a food processor. Pulse until thoroughly mixed. 3. Transfer the mixture onto a baking sheet and shape it into falafel patties. 4. Brush each falafel with olive oil and bake for 20 to 25 minutes or until golden brown. 5. Serve the baked sweet potato and chickpea falafel with tahini sauce.

10. Caprese Chicken Skillet

Prep Time: 10 minutes | Cooking Time: 20 minutes

Ingredients	Instruction
- 4 skinless, boneless chicken breasts	1. Sprinkle salt and pepper on the chicken breasts.
- 1 tablespoon olive oil	2. Heat olive oil in a big skillet over medium-high heat.
- 1/2 cup diced fresh mozzarella	3. Add chicken breasts and until browned on both sides and cooked through.
- 2 tablespoons balsamic vinegar	4. Place cherry tomatoes, fresh mozzarella, and balsamic vinegar in the same skillet.
- 1 tablespoon chopped fresh basil	5. Simmer until the cheese has melted and the tomatoes are softened.
- Salt and pepper to taste	6. Before serving, garnish with fresh basil.

Feel free to modify these recipes to suit your own tastes and any specific blood type considerations. Enjoy these delicious and wholesome dinner options on the Blood Type AB Positive Diet!

1. Almond Butter and Banana Protein Bites

Prep Time: 15 minutes | Chilling Time: 1 hour

Ingredients	Instruction
- 1 cup almond butter - 1 mashed ripe banana - 1/4 cup chia seeds - 1/4 cup flaxseed meal - 1/4 cup honey - 1/2 cup shredded coconut (optional for coating) - 1 teaspoon vanilla extract - A pinch of sea salt	1. Combine almond butter, mashed banana, flaxseed meal, chia seeds, honey, vanilla extract, and a pinch of sea salt in a bowl. 2. Mix until thoroughly combined. 3. To firm up the mixture, refrigerate for 30 minutes. 4. Scoop out tiny bits and form into bite-sized balls. 5. Roll the balls in shredded coconut for added texture, if desired 6. Before serving, refrigerate for an extra 30 minutes.

2. Berry and Yogurt Parfait

Prep Time: 10 minutes | Assembly Time: 5 minutes

Ingredients	Instruction
- 1 cup Greek yogurt - 1/2 cup mixed berries (raspberries, strawberries, and blueberries) - 1/4 cup granola - 1 tablespoon honey - 1/4 teaspoon vanilla extract	1. Layer Greek yogurt at the bottom of a glass or bowl. 2. Top the yogurt with a layer of mixed berries. 3. Evenly sprinkle granola on top of the berries. 4. Pour vanilla extract and honey on top of the granola. 5. Continue layering until the bowl or glass is full. 6. Serve immediately as a nutrient-rich, refreshing parfait.

3. Dark Chocolate Avocado Mousse

Prep Time: 10 minutes | Chilling Time: 1 hour

Ingredients	Instruction
- 1/4 cup unsweetened cocoa powder - 2 ripe avocados, peeled and pitted - 1/4 cup maple syrup - 1 teaspoon vanilla extract -Pinch of sea salt - Dark chocolate shavings for garnish, if desired	1. Combine avocados, cocoa powder, maple syrup, vanilla extract, and pinch of sea salt in a blender or food processor. 2. Blend until creamy and smooth. 3. Refrigerate the mousse for at least 1 hour to chill. 4. Transfer the cooled mousse into dishes for serving. 5. If preferred, garnish with dark chocolate shavings. 6. As a decadent and rich dessert, serve cold.

4. Apple and Almond Butter Nachos

Prep Time: 10 minutes | Assembly Time: 5 minutes

Ingredients	Instruction
- 2 thinly sliced and cored apples	1. Place the apple slices in a circular pattern on a plate.
- 1/4 cup almond butter	2. For easy drizzling, slightly warm the almond butter.
- 2 tablespoons chopped almonds	3. Drizzle almond butter over apple slices.
- 1 tablespoon coconut, shredded	4. Top with shredded coconut and chopped almonds.
- 1 tablespoon honey	5. Pour honey on top of the nachos.
- Cinnamon for sprinkling	6. Add a sprinkle of cinnamon.
	7. Serve right away as a filling and crunchy snack.

5. Chia Seed Pudding with Mixed Berries

Prep Time: 5 minutes | Chilling Time: 2 hours or overnight

Ingredients	Instruction
- 1/4 cup chia seeds - 1 cup almond milk - 1/4 teaspoon vanilla extract - 1/2 cup mixed berries (strawberries, raspberries, and blueberries) - 1 tablespoon honey	1. Combine almond milk, honey, vanilla extract, and chia seeds in a bowl. 2. Stir well, then freeze for at least 2 hours or overnight. 3. Give the chia pudding a thorough stir after it has set. 4. Ladle the chia pudding into glasses or serving bowls. 5. Before serving, sprinkle mixed berries over top. 6. Savor this tasty and nutrient-rich chia seed pudding.

6. Apple and Almond Butter Sandwiches

Prep Time: 5 minutes

Ingredients	Instruction
- 2 medium apples, cored and sliced into rounds - Almonds butter - Granola - Chia seeds - Maple syrup or honey	1. On one side of the apple slices, spread almond butter. 2. Sprinkle granola and chia seeds on the almond butter. 3. To make a sandwich, place another apple slice on top. 4. If preferred, drizzle with maple syrup or honey. 5. Serve right away for a tasty and crunchy snack.

7. Mango and Coconut Chia Pudding

Prep Time: 15 minutes | Chilling Time: 1 hour

Ingredients	Instruction
- 1/4 cup chia seeds - 1 cup dairy or non-dairy milk - 1 diced ripe mango - 2 tablespoons shredded coconut - 1 tablespoon sweetener (honey, maple syrup, or agave nectar) - Fresh mint for garnish	1. Combine milk and chia seeds in a bowl. Allow it to sit for 10 minutes, stirring occasionally. 2. Layer mango slices in the base of serving glasses. 3. Drizzle the mango with the chia seed mixture. 4. Sprinkle shredded coconut on top. 5. Garnish with fresh mint and drizzle with sweetener. 6. Before serving, Freeze for at least 1 hour.

8. Nutty Banana Bites

Prep Time: 5 minutes

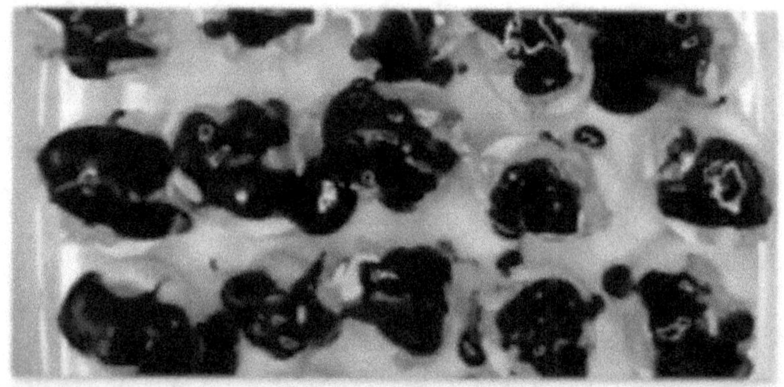

Ingredients	Instruction
- 2 sliced bananas - Peanut butter or almond butter - Chopped nuts (pistachios, walnuts, or almonds) - Cinnamon - Dark chocolate chips	1. Apply peanut butter or almond butter to the banana slices. 2. Add a pinch of cinnamon and chopped nuts. 3. Top with dark chocolate chips. 4. Serve right away for a tasty and speedy snack.

9. Almond and Coconut Energy Bars

Prep Time: 15 minutes | Chilling Time: 2 hours

Ingredients	Instruction
- 1 cup almonds - 1 cup coconut, shredded - 1/2 cup dates, pitted - 1/4 cup protein powder - 2 tablespoons almond butter - 1 tablespoon sweetener (honey, maple syrup, agave nectar) - A dash of salt	1.　Blend almonds, shredded coconut, pitted dates, protein powder, almond butter, sweetener, and a dash of salt in a food processor. 2. Process the ingredients until a sticky dough forms. 3. Transfer the mixture to a lined baking dish, and then freeze for at least 2 hours. 4. Cut into bars and savor these nutrient-packed energy bars.

10. Chilled Berry Soup

Prep Time: 10 minutes | Chilling Time: 1 hour

Ingredients	Instruction
- 2 cups mixed berries (strawberries, blueberries, raspberries) - 1 cup yogurt (dairy or non-dairy) - 1 tablespoon sweetener (honey, maple syrup, agave nectar) - 1/2 teaspoon vanilla extract - Fresh mint for garnish	1. Combine mixed berries, yogurt, sweetener, and vanilla extract in a blender. 2. Blend until smooth. 3. Freeze the berry soup for at least 1 hour. 4. Before serving, garnish with fresh mint. 5. For a cool, guilt-free dessert, serve chilled.

Adapt these recipes to your own tastes and any particular blood type that may apply. Enjoy these delightful and nutritious snacks and desserts on the Blood Type AB Positive Diet!

Smoothie with Boost

1. Berry Bliss Smoothie

Prep Time: 5 minutes | Blending Time: 2 minutes

Ingredients	Instruction
- 1 cup mixed berries (strawberries, raspberries, blueberries) - 1/2 cup dairy or non-dairy yogurt - 1/2 cup milk (soy, almond, or coconut) - 1 tablespoon chia seeds - 1 tablespoon almond butter - 1 teaspoon honey or maple syrup, if preferred - Ice cubes	1. Combine yogurt, milk, chia seeds, almond butter, mixed berries, and honey (if using) in a blender. 2. Process until smooth's 3. Add ice cubes and blend again until well combined. 4. Pour into a glass and enjoy this refreshing Berry Bliss Smoothie.

2. Green Goddess Smoothie

Prep Time: 7 minutes | Blending Time: 3 minutes

Ingredients	Instruction
- 1 cup spinach leaves - 1/2 cup sliced cucumber - 1/2 avocado (peeled and pitted) - 1/2 banana - 1 cup milk (soy, coconut, or almond) - 1 tablespoon chia seeds - Fresh mint leaves for decoration - Ice cubes	1. Combine spinach, cucumber, avocado, banana, milk, and chia seeds in a blender. 2. Process until smooth. 3. Add ice cubes and process again to obtain the required consistency. 4. Transfer into a glass and add some fresh mint leaves as a garnish. 5. Enjoy this nutrient-packed Green Goddess Smoothie.

3. Tropical Paradise Smoothie

Prep Time: 6 minutes | Blending Time: 2 minutes

Ingredients	Instruction
- Half a cup of chopped pineapple - 1/2 cup chunky mango - 1/2 banana - 1/2 cup dairy-free or dairy yogurt - 1/2 cup milk (soy, almond, or coconut) - 1 tablespoon coconut, shredded - 1 teaspoon honey or maple syrup, if desired - Cubes of ice	1. Combine banana, pineapple, mango, yogurt, milk, shredded coconut, and honey (if using) in a blender. 2. Process until smooth. 3. Add the ice cubes and Blend again to obtain the desired consistency. 4. Transfer the Tropical Paradise Smoothie into a glass and enjoy.

4. Protein-Packed Almond Delight

Prep Time: 5 minutes | Blending Time: 3 minutes

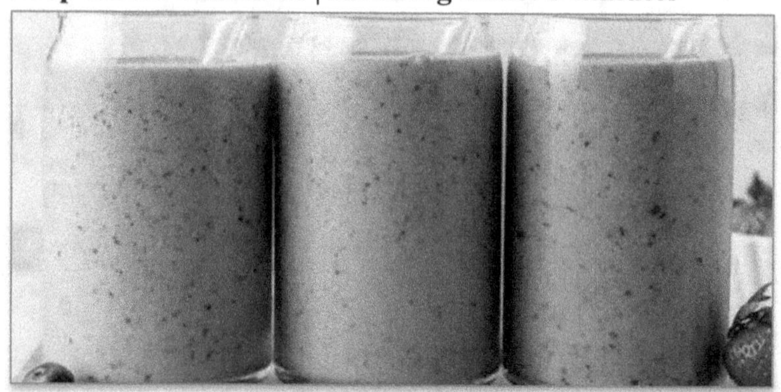

Ingredients	Instruction
- 1 cup milk (soy, coconut, or almond) - 1/2 banana - 1/4 cup almonds - 1 tablespoon almond butter - One scoop (vegetable-based) protein powder - 1 teaspoon chia seeds - Ice cubes	1. Combine milk, banana, almond butter, chia seeds, protein powder, and almonds in a blender. 2. Blend until smooth. 3. Add the ice cubes and blend again to obtain the desired consistency. 4. Transfer into a glass and savor the Protein-Packed Almond Delight.

5. Citrus Burst Smoothie

Prep Time: 6 minutes | Blending Time: 2 minutes

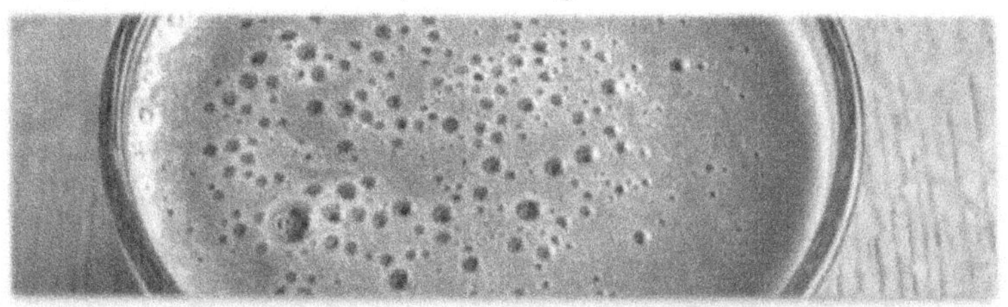

Ingredients	Instruction
- 1 orange, peeled and segmented - 1/2 cup (dairy-free or dairy) yogurt - 1/2 cup milk (soy, almond, or coconut) - 1/2 banana - 1 tablespoon chia seeds - 1 teaspoon honey or maple syrup, if desired - Ice cubes	1. Combine orange segments, yogurt, milk, banana, chia seeds, and honey (if using) in a blender. 2. Blend until smooth. 3. Add ice cubes and blend again to obtain the required consistency. 4. Transfer to a glass and relish the Citrus Burst Smoothie.

6. Blueberry Bliss Smoothie

Prep Time: 5 minutes | Blending Time: 2 minutes

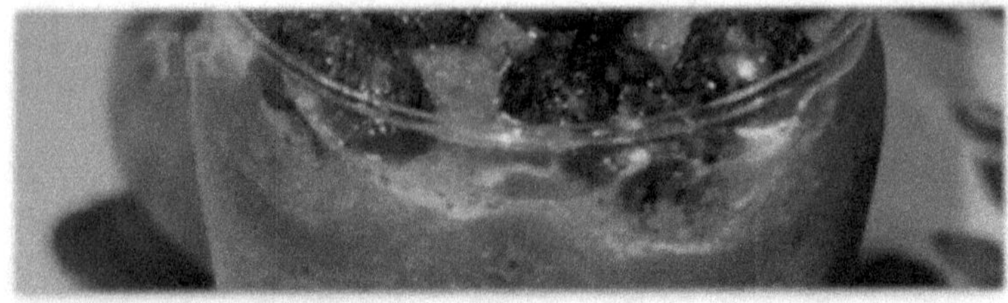

Ingredients	Instruction
- 1 cup (frozen or fresh) blueberries - 1/2 cup dairy-free or dairy yogurt - 1/2 cup milk (soy, almond, coconut) - 1 tablespoon almond butter - 1 tablespoon flaxseeds - 1 teaspoon honey or maple syrup if desired - Ice cubes	1. Combine almond butter, blueberries, yogurt, milk, flaxseeds, and honey (if using) in a blender. 2. Blend until smooth. 3. Add ice cubes and blend again to obtain the required consistency. 4. Transfer into a glass and relish the blissful Blueberry Smoothie.

7. Spinach and Pineapple Delight

Prep Time: 6 minutes | Blending Time: 3 minutes

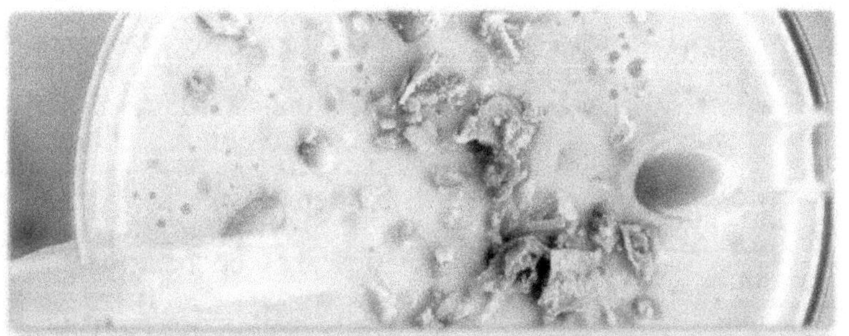

Ingredients	Instruction
- 1 cup fresh spinach - 1/2 cup pineapple chunks - 1/2 banana - 1/2 cup dairy-free or dairy yogurt - 1/2 cup milk (soy, almond, coconut) - 1 tablespoon chia seeds - Ice cubes	1. Combine spinach, banana, pineapple, yogurt, milk, and chia seeds in a blender. 2. Blend until smooth. 3. Add ice cubes and blend again to obtain the required consistency. 4. Transfer to a glass and savor the Spinach and Pineapple Delight.

8. Chocolate Banana Protein Shake

Prep Time: 5 minutes | Blending Time: 2 minutes

Ingredients	Instruction
- 1 banana - 1 cup blood milk (almond, coconut, or soy) - 2 teaspoons (vegetable-based) protein powder - 1 tablespoon powdered cocoa - 1 tablespoon almond butter - 1 teaspoon honey or maple syrup, if desired - Ice cubes	1. Combine almond butter, banana, protein powder, cocoa powder, milk, and honey (if using) in a blender. 2. Blend until smooth. 3. Add ice cubes and blend once more to obtain the required consistency. 4. Transfer the Chocolate Banana Protein Shake into a glass and enjoy.

9. Raspberry Coconut Refresher

Prep Time: 6 minutes | Blending Time: 3 minutes

Ingredients	Instruction
- 1 cup (frozen or fresh) raspberries - 1/2 cup coconut milk - 1/2 cup (non-dairy or dairy) yogurt - 1 tablespoon shredded coconut - 1 tablespoon chia seeds - 1 teaspoon honey or maple syrup, if desired - Ice cubes	1. Combine raspberries, yogurt, chia seeds, shredded coconut, coconut milk, and honey (if using) in a blender. 2. Blend until smooth. 3. Add ice cubes and blend once more to obtain the required consistency. 4. Pour the Raspberry Coconut Refresher into a glass and enjoy.

10. Kiwi and Mint Citrus Smoothie

Prep Time: 7 minutes

Ingredients	Instruction
- 2 peeled and sliced kiwis - 1/2 cup orange juice - 1/2 cup yogurt, (dairy or non-dairy) - 1 tablespoon fresh mint leaves - 1 tablespoon chia seeds - 1 teaspoon honey or maple syrup, if desired - Ice cubes	1. Combine kiwis, yogurt, orange juice, chia seeds, mint leaves, and honey (if using) in a blender. 2. Blend until smooth. 3. Add ice cubes and blend once more to obtain the required consistency. 4. Transfer the Kiwi and Mint Citrus Smoothie into a glass and savor it.

7-day Meal Plan for Blood Type AB+ Individuals

Breakfast: Berry Bliss Smoothie

Lunch: Quinoa Salad with Grilled Chicken

Snack: Apple and Almond Butter Quesadillas

Dinner: Baked Lemon Herb Chicken

Breakfast: Green Goddess Smoothie

Lunch: Mediterranean Chickpea Salad

Snack: Mango and Avocado Salsa

Dinner: Stir-Fried Tofu with Vegetables

Breakfast: Chocolate Banana Protein Shake

Lunch: Turkey and Spinach Stuffed Mushrooms

Snack: Pumpkin Chia Seed Pudding

Dinner: Quinoa and Black Bean Stuffed Peppers

DAY 4:

Breakfast: Raspberry Coconut Refresher

Lunch: Caprese Chicken Skillet

Snack: Blueberry and Mint Sorbet

Dinner: Sweet Potato and Chickpea Coconut Curry

DAY 5:

Breakfast: Kiwi and Mint Citrus Smoothie

Lunch: Baked Sweet Potato and Chickpea Falafel

Snack: Almond Butter Banana Bites

Dinner: Lemon Herb Quinoa with Grilled Shrimp

DAY 6:

Breakfast: Blueberry Bliss Smoothie

Lunch: Lentil and Vegetable Stir-Fry

Snack: Mango and Berry Yogurt Parfait

Dinner: Grilled Salmon with Lemon Dill Sauce

DAY 7:

Breakfast: Spinach and Pineapple Delight

Lunch: Greek Salad with Grilled Chicken

Snack: Chocolate Avocado Mousse

Dinner: Vegetable and Chickpea Coconut Curry

Feel free to adjust portion sizes and ingredients based on individual preferences and dietary needs. This meal plan provides a variety of flavors and nutrients to support the Blood Type AB+ individual's well-being.

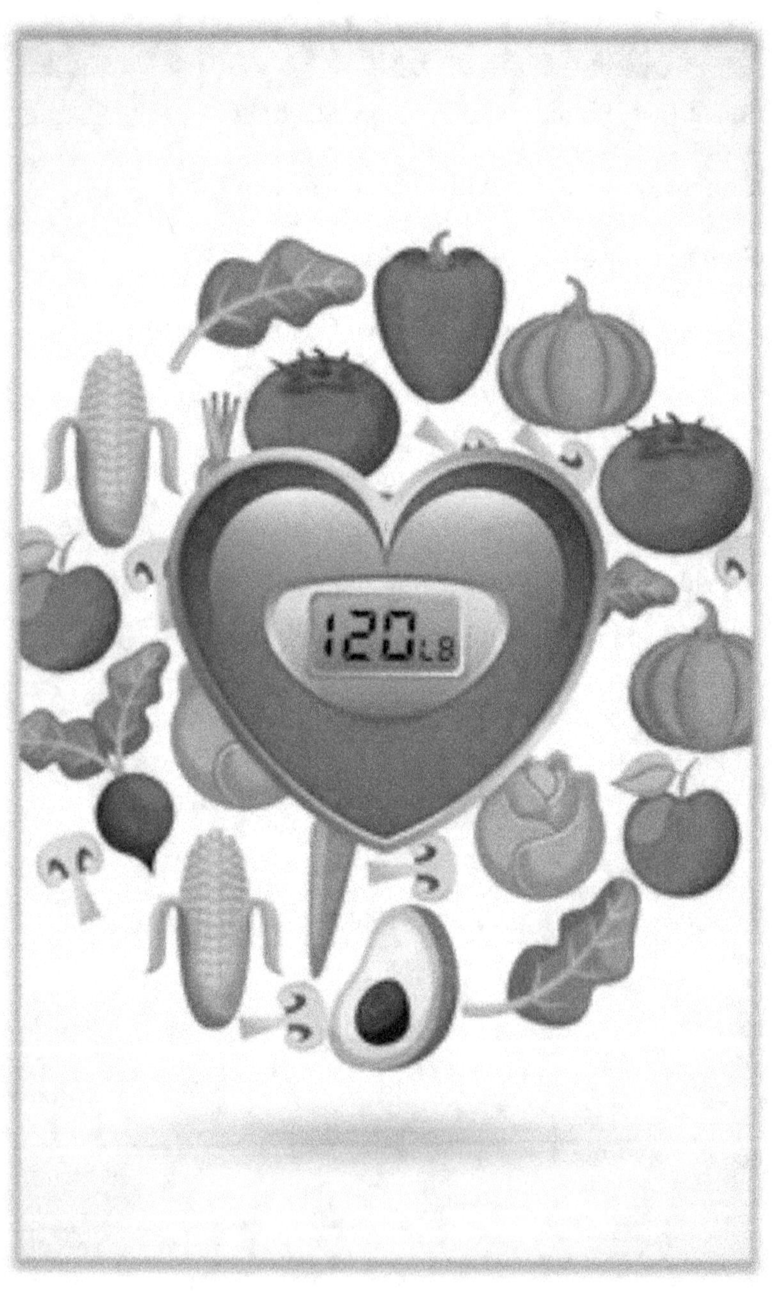

120 LB

Conclusion

To sum up, the **Blood Type AB-Positive Diet Book** seeks to equip you with the information and resources necessary to adopt a customized and all-encompassing approach to healthy living. Through insightful guidance on blood type-specific nutrition, this book has explored the unique characteristics, nutritional needs, and meal options specifically beneficial for those with Blood Type AB-Positive.

Understanding the subtleties of this blood type has helped us create a wide variety of meals, from healthy dinners and snacks to delicious smoothies and stimulating breakfasts. Incorporating blood type-friendly products such as grains, fruits, vegetables, and proteins guarantees mouthwatering flavors and promotes general health.

Adopting this dietary strategy can help you achieve optimal health, which may include improved digestion, energy levels, and metabolism. The carefully selected menus and recipes provide a well-rounded nutritional profile while accounting for the unique needs of blood type AB-Positive individuals.

Remember that following the Blood Type AB-Positive Diet is a step towards long-term well-being, not just a temporary commitment, as you set out on this path towards a healthier living. Your body is unique, and by aligning your diet with your blood type, you are customizing your approach to nutrition, potentially unlocking the key to a healthier, more vibrant life.

You are investing in your own health and vigor by consciously choosing to follow and adjust to this diet. Let the joy of preparing and savoring these blood type-conscious meals become a celebration of self-care. Your dedication to this individualized method has the potential to completely improve your overall health as well as your nutrition. Embrace the journey, relish the flavors, and witness the positive impact on your health as you embark on the path to a more vibrant and healthier you. Your body, after all, deserves the very best.

Cheers to a nourished and thriving life!

Thank you for purchasing and choosing to embark on this culinary adventure with us. *Your support and readership are deeply appreciated.*

Could you please leave us a review? Your honest feedback is not only invaluable but crucial in shaping our future endeavors.

By leaving a review, you not only help us understand what resonates with you but also empower fellow readers to make informed decisions and help this books reach more potential readers. Also consider recommending it to friends or family who share your interest. Your words have the power to inspire and guide others.

Thank you for being part of this journey, we look forward hearing from you.

Kindly open your phone camera and place it on the barcode to scan.

It will link you directly to the review page.

Scan the QR code below to get more books from

the author

Weekly Meal Planner Journal

Date: _____________

DAYS	BREAKFAST	LUNCH	DINNER
MON			
TUE			
WED			
THU			
FRI			
SAT			
SUN			

Shopping List

- _______________________
- _______________________
- _______________________
- _______________________

NOTES

Weekly Meal Planner Journal

Date: _______________

DAYS	BREAKFAST	LUNCH	DINNER
MON			
TUE			
WED			
THU			
FRI			
SAT			
SUN			

Shopping List

- _______________________________
- _______________________________
- _______________________________
- _______________________________

NOTES

Weekly Meal Planner Journal

Date: _______________

DAYS	BREAKFAST	LUNCH	DINNER
MON			
TUE			
WED			
THU			
FRI			
SAT			
SUN			

Shopping List

- _______________
- _______________
- _______________
- _______________

NOTES

Weekly Meal Planner Journal

Date: ___________

DAYS	BREAKFAST	LUNCH	DINNER
MON			
TUE			
WED			
THU			
FRI			
SAT			
SUN			

Shopping List

- ___________________________________
- ___________________________________
- ___________________________________
- ___________________________________

NOTES

Weekly Meal Planner Journal

Date: _______________

DAYS	BREAKFAST	LUNCH	DINNER
MON			
TUE			
WED			
THU			
FRI			
SAT			
SUN			

Shopping List

- _______________________________
- _______________________________
- _______________________________
- _______________________________

NOTES

Weekly Meal Planner Journal

Date: _______________

DAYS	BREAKFAST	LUNCH	DINNER
MON			
TUE			
WED			
THU			
FRI			
SAT			
SUN			

Shopping List

- ____
- ____
- ____
- ____

NOTES

Weekly Meal Planner Journal

Date: ___________

DAYS	BREAKFAST	LUNCH	DINNER
MON			
TUE			
WED			
THU			
FRI			
SAT			
SUN			

Shopping List

- ____________________________
- ____________________________
- ____________________________
- ____________________________

NOTES

Weekly Meal Planner Journal

Date: ______________

DAYS	BREAKFAST	LUNCH	DINNER
MON			
TUE			
WED			
THU			
FRI			
SAT			
SUN			

Shopping List

- ____
- ____
- ____
- ____

NOTES

Weekly Meal Planner Journal

Date: _______________

DAYS	BREAKFAST	LUNCH	DINNER
MON			
TUE			
WED			
THU			
FRI			
SAT			
SUN			

Shopping List

- _______________________________________
- _______________________________________
- _______________________________________
- _______________________________________

NOTES

Weekly Meal Planner Journal

Date: _____________

DAYS	BREAKFAST	LUNCH	DINNER
MON			
TUE			
WED			
THU			
FRI			
SAT			
SUN			

Shopping List

- ____
- ____
- ____
- ____

NOTES